What people are saying:

Picture Memories – Understanding Dementia is a beautifully written book that explains Alzheimer's disease in a most sensitive manner. The Henderson family's understanding of the needs of family members facing this diagnosis for children with intellectual disabilities is impressive and their ability to communicate what the disease means is nothing short of phenomenal! The book is breathtakingly beautiful and will help any family dealing with this diagnosis. It is a must read.

Suzanne Sewell
President & CEO
Florida ARF

It made me cry - and it made me smile, both of which are crucial for a reader in order to get the full impact of the book's meaning. I think it is a clear explanation for people of all ages - even those of us who think we understand this disease because we know the medical facts; this goes beyond the facts of the body and brings home the facts of the heart. I see this book as helping not only families whose loved one has Down syndrome, but all families facing this new journey. Thanks to Trey and the Hendersons for sharing so much of their own lives in order to bring information and encouragement to the lives of so many others.

Laura Watts
Co-foundeer
Jacksonville Down
Syndrome Assiciation

Although originally written to help the patient, this well written, easy to understand and beautifully illustrated book can help others, especially young family members, better empathize with a loved one who is suffering from dementia. It will be an essential addition to my own bookshelf.

Dr. Joseph Sarachene, MD
Physiologist

Picture Memories – Understanding Dementia is a beautiful and touching book providing an understanding of Alzheimer's and dementia. This poignant, well written and illustrated book gives an explanation in simplistic terms and provides insight to families who are struggling to understand and cope with dementia and Alzheimer's.

Leslie Weed
Co-Founder
HEAL Foundation

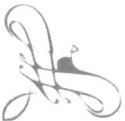

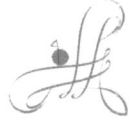

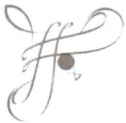

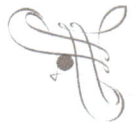

Picture Memories
UNDERSTANDING
DEMENTIA

SHERRI HENDERSON

Illustrated by
ANI BARMASHI

Foreword written by
DR. LINDA EDWARDS, MD

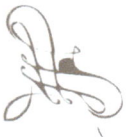

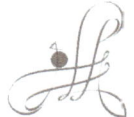

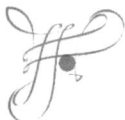

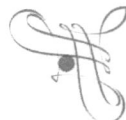

Picture Memories - Understanding Dementia
By Sherri Henderson

For permission requests, write to the publisher, Attention: Permissions Coordinator, at the address below:

Henderson Haven, Inc.
772 Foxridge Center Dr.
Orange Park, FL 32065
www.HendersonHaven.org

Ordering information: Quantity sales. Special discounts are available on quantity purchases by corporations, associations, and others. For details, contact the publisher at the address above.

Printed in the United States of America

LCCN: 2018936222
ISBN: 978-1-7320118-0-9

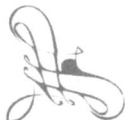

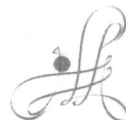

How often do we use the phrase "a picture is worth a thousand words"? Imagine trying to explain to a young adult with Down syndrome and intellectual disability the reason their memory is declining. We know that persons with Down syndrome are more likely to experience dementia, but nothing prepares parents, caregivers and loved ones for this devastating reality when it happens. Perhaps the most troubling aspect of all is that the young adult with dementia may not be able to share what they are thinking: what they fear, what they do or do not understand. The author has offered a thoughtful approach she and her family are using to talk with their son about this new chapter in his and their lives.

Dementia, or loss of "picture memories", as is so eloquently described by the author, affects over 5% of adults over the age of 65. Although this book has been written to help young adults who are beginning to lose their picture memories, families, caregivers, loved ones and physicians can learn from this simple but eloquent description of dementia. The phrase "picture memories" will forever be on my mind when I am talking with patients and their loved ones about dementia, regardless of their age. I am thankful to the author and illustrator for their simple but beautiful book to help young adults with fading memory understand and adapt to this new chapter in their lives.

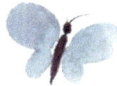

Dr. Linda R. Edwards, M.D.

Senior Associate Dean for Educational Affairs; Chief, Division of General Internal Medicine; Associate Chair, Department of Medicine; Medical Director, Program for Adults with Intellectual and Developmental Disabilities UF Health Shands, Jacksonville, FL

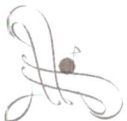

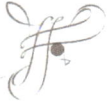

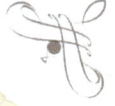

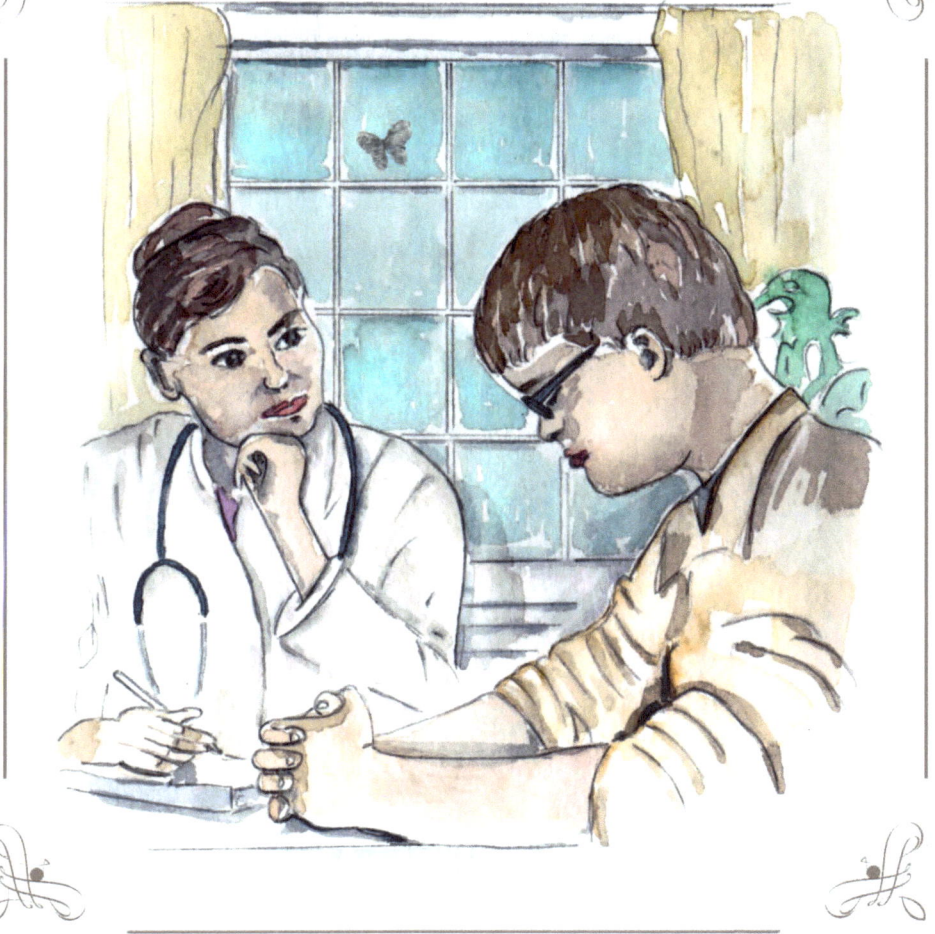

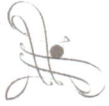

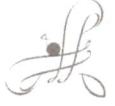

"You have Alzheimer's,"
the doctor says.

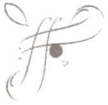

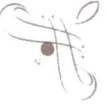

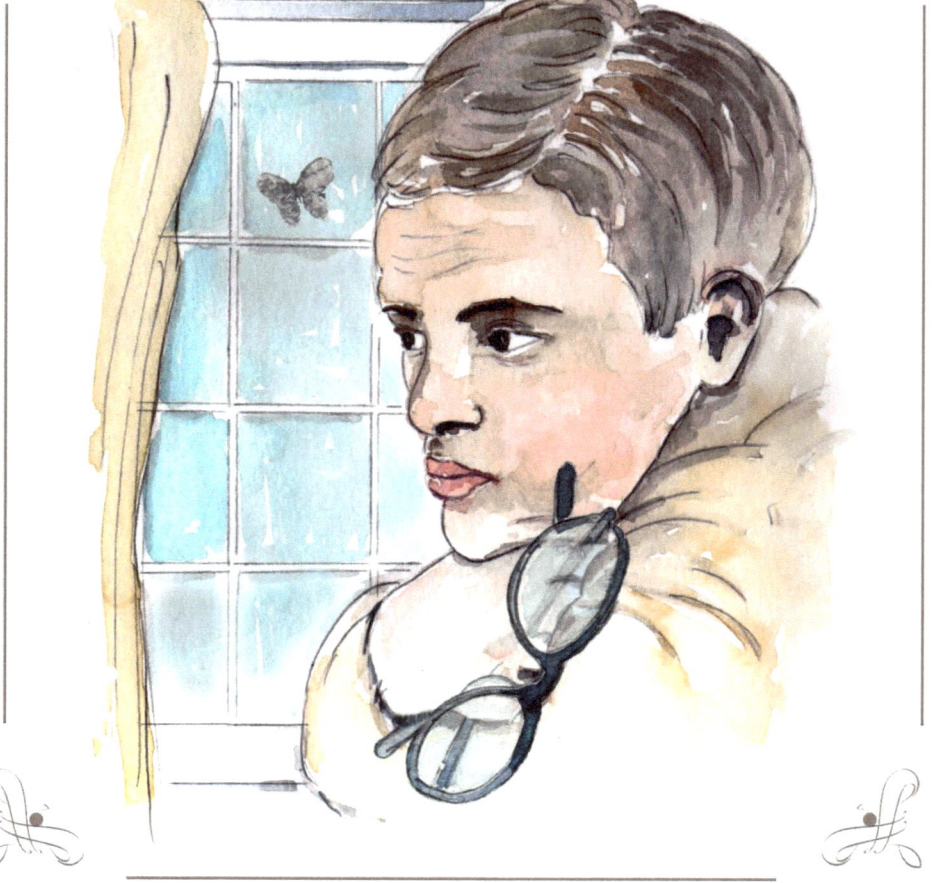

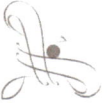

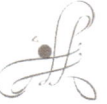

So what does that mean?

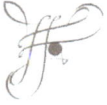

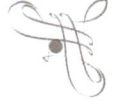

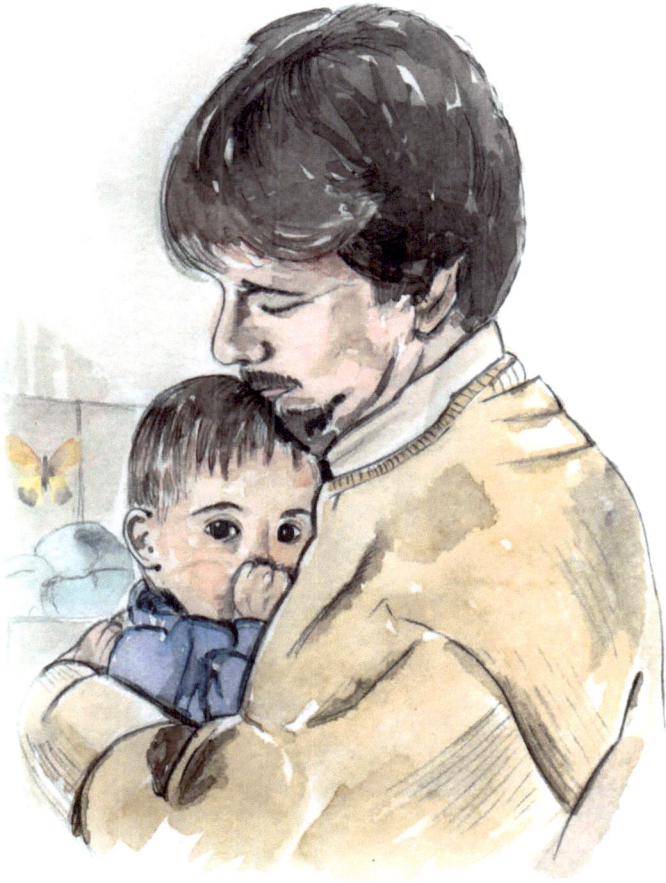

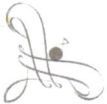

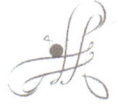

Let's start when we're small.

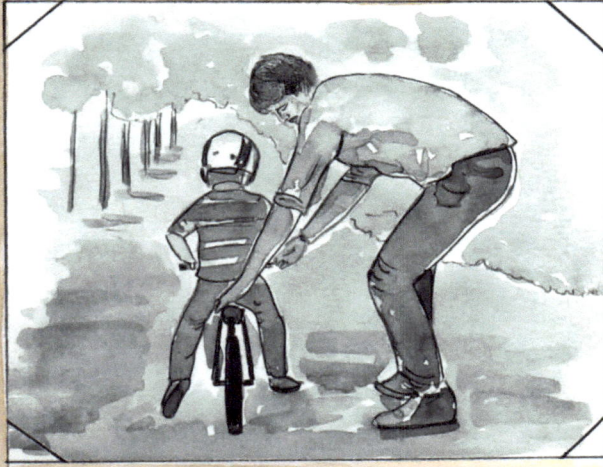

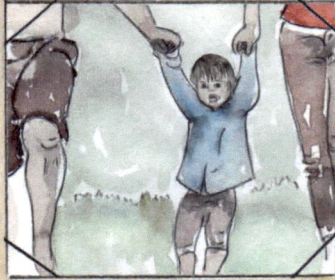

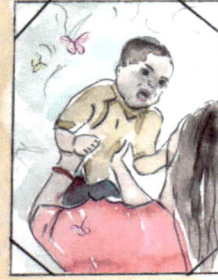

Our brain begins to take pictures of
people, places and things important in
our lives.

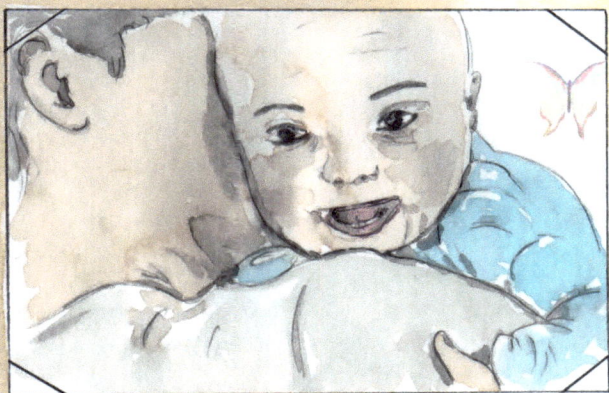

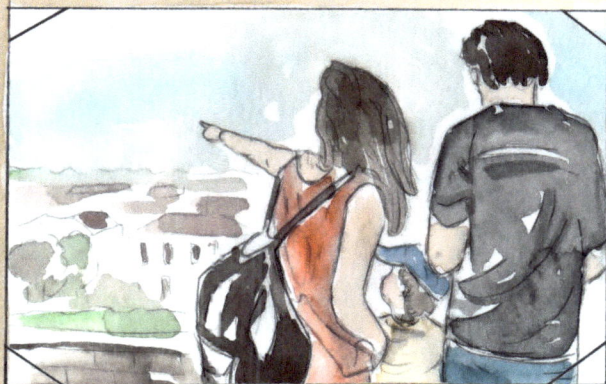

They are the very best pictures.
We keep them in our hearts and minds
to remember.

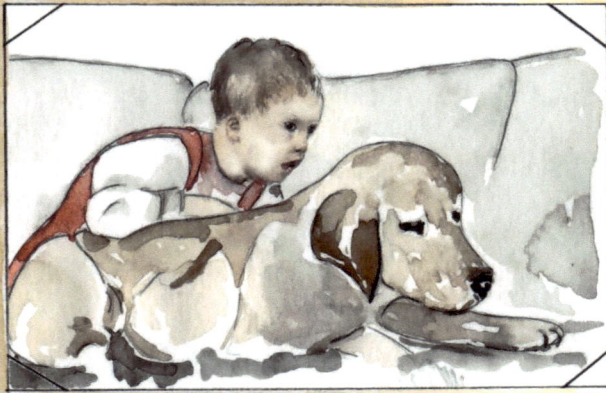

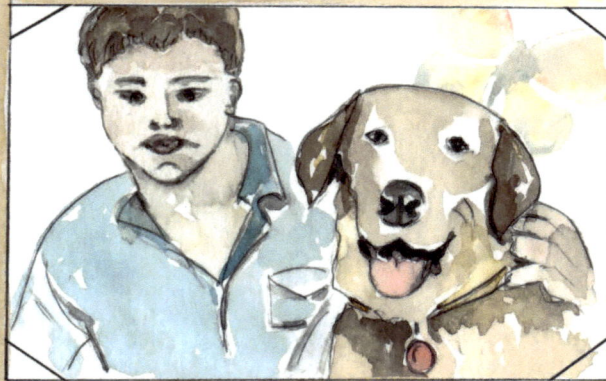

Every day for the rest of our lives,
our brain keeps taking these
picture memories.

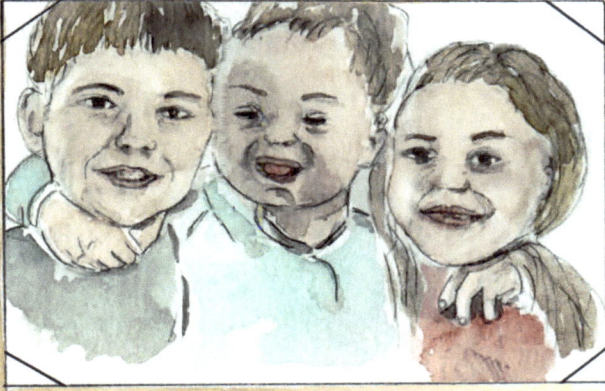

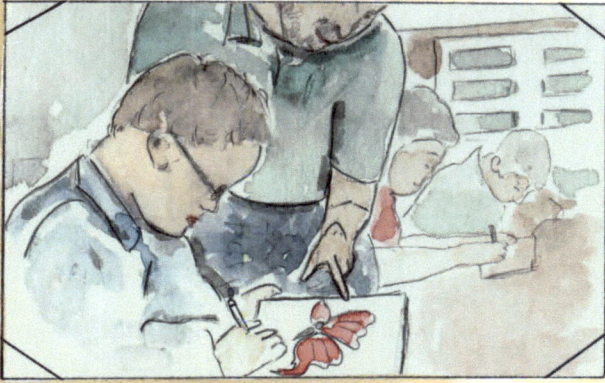

Some pictures help us
remember people and places
important to us.

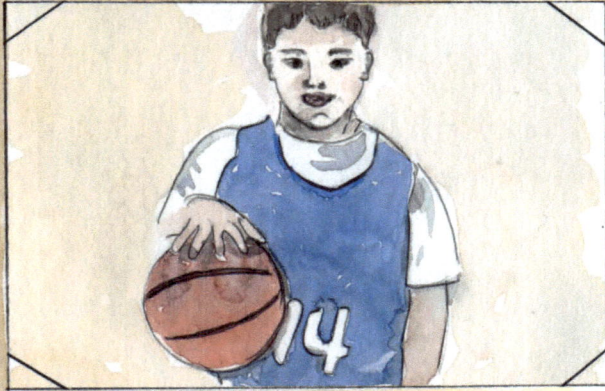

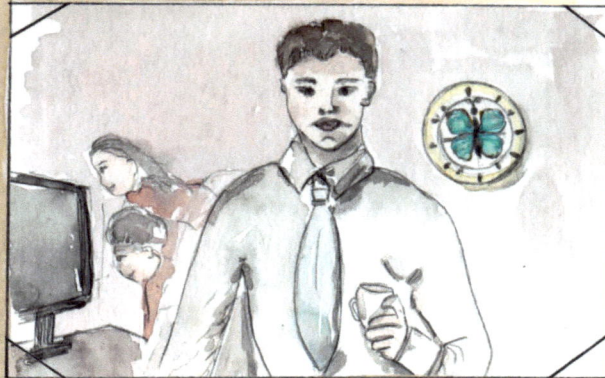

Some help us to remember
how to do things.

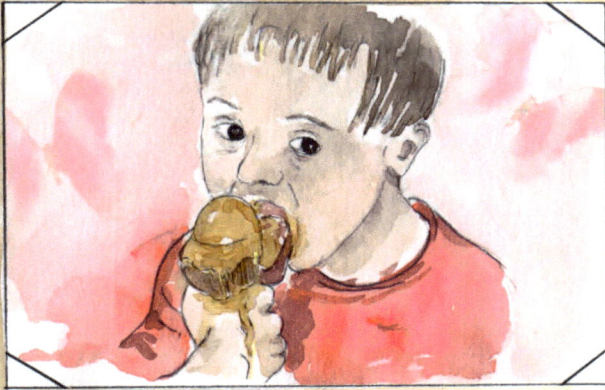

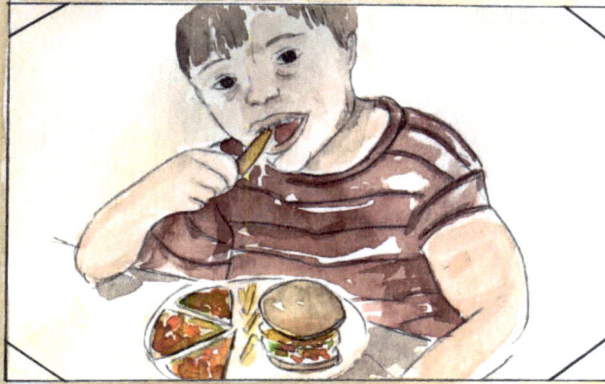

Some picture memories
remind us what foods we like.

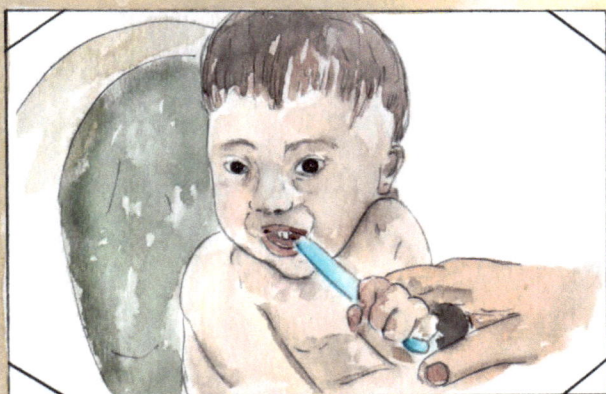

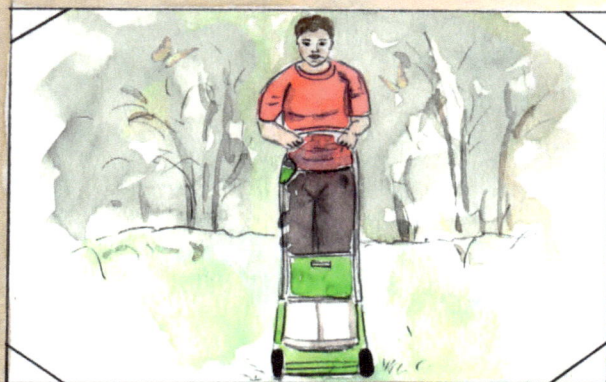

And some remind us
how to take care of ourselves.

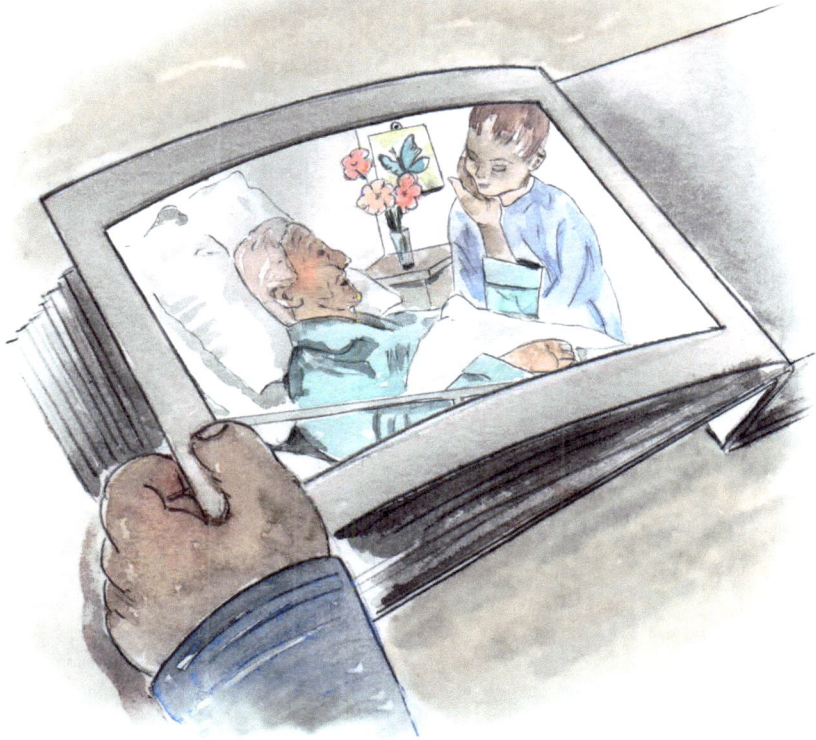

Some picture memories
make us sad,

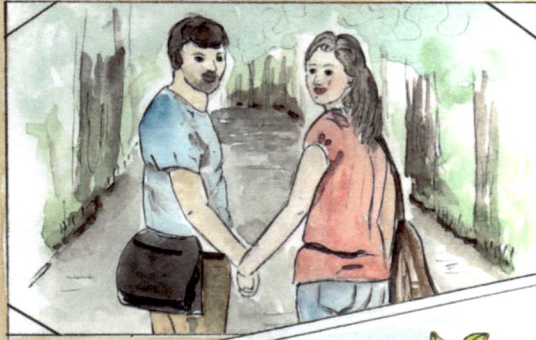

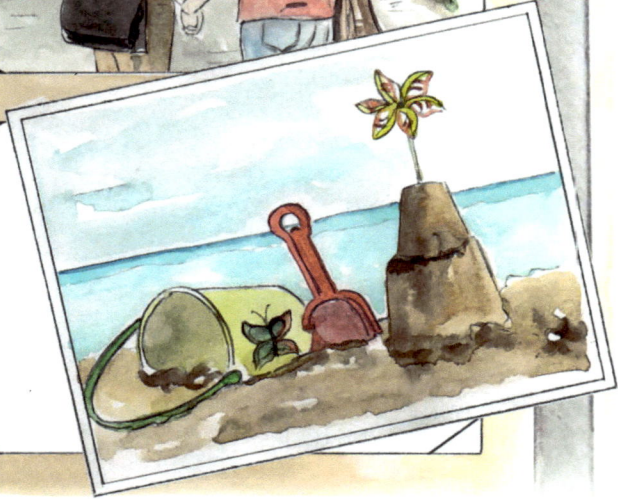

but even more make us
really happy to remember.

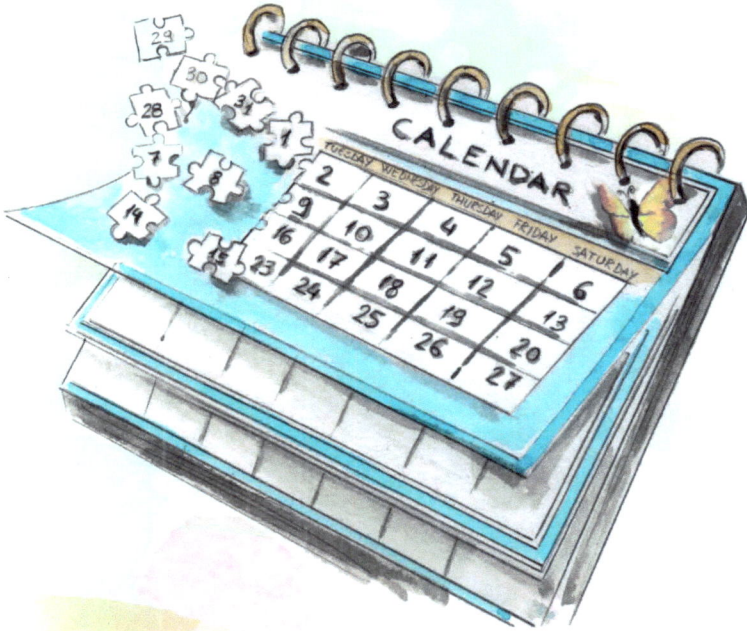

When the doctor tells us
we have Alzheimer's or dementia,
some of our picture memories
have already started to fade.

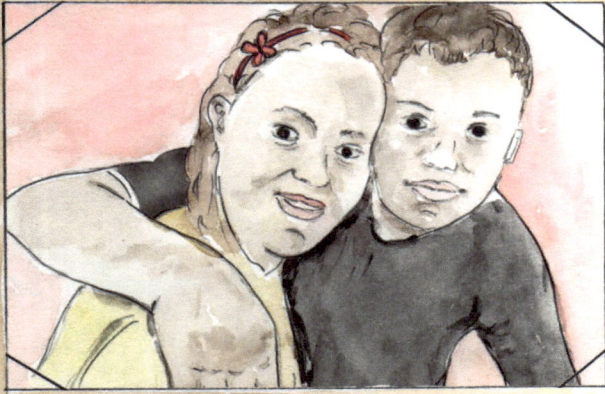

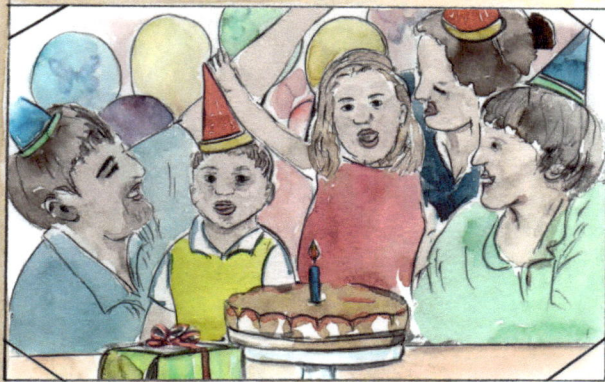

Sometimes, the easiest
pictures to find are often
the ones we took first.

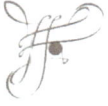

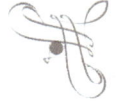

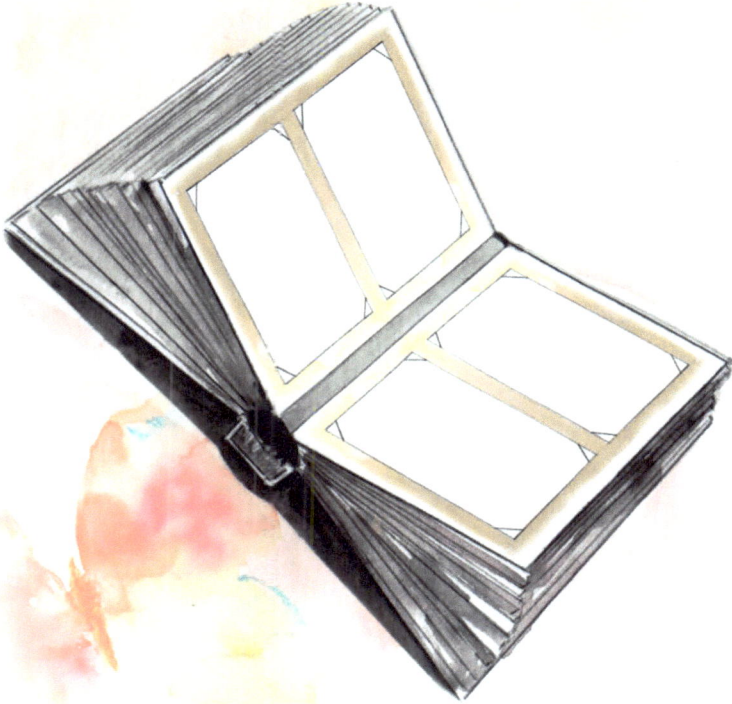

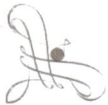

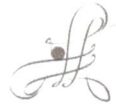

Some days, our brain will forget
to take pictures,or we may not
be able to find them at all.

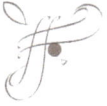

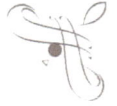

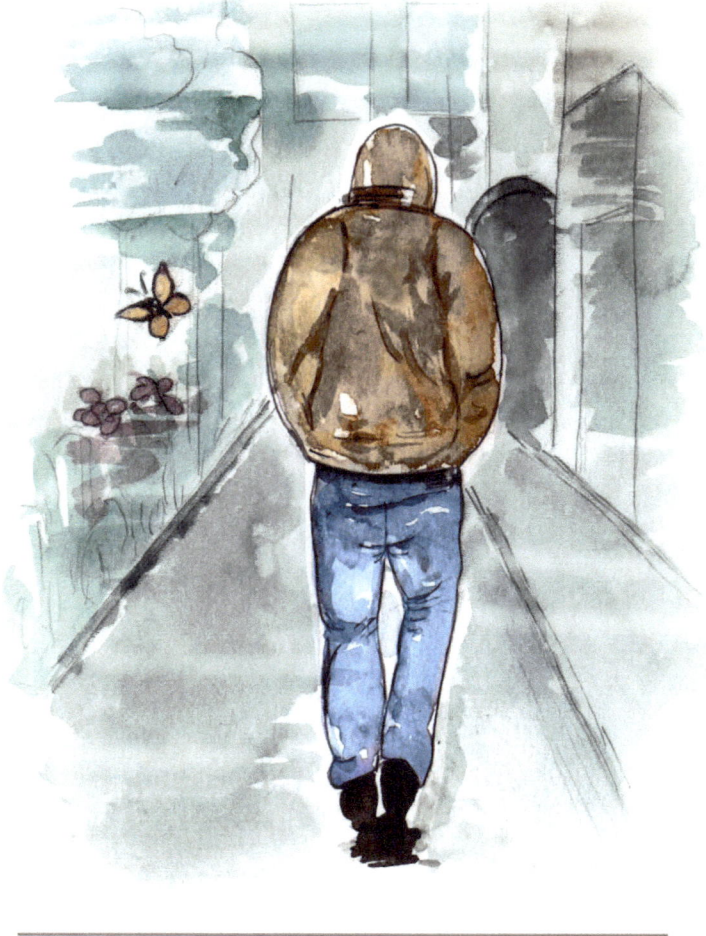

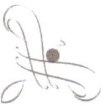

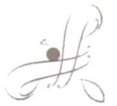

When that happens,
we may forget how to get home;

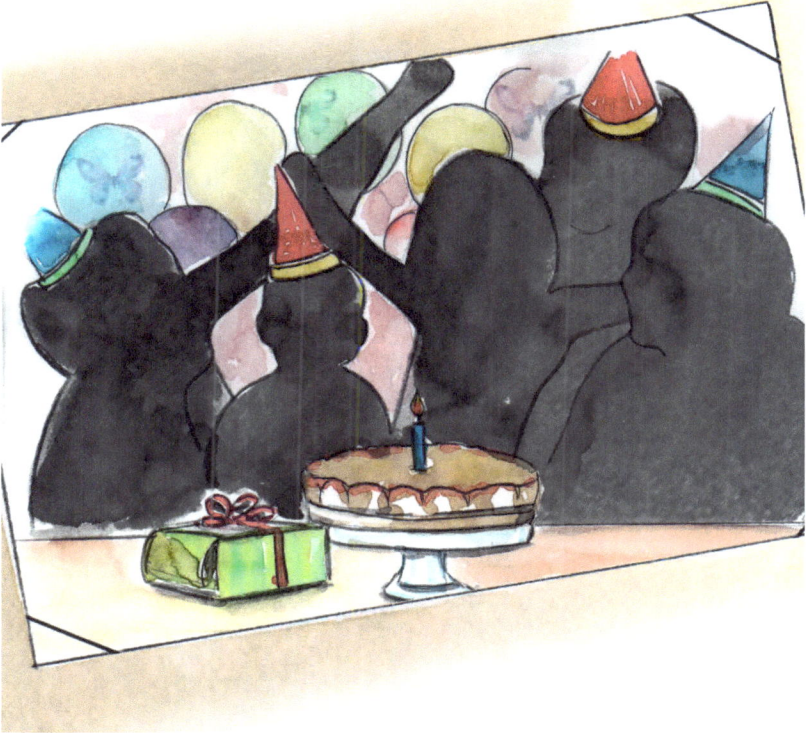

we may forget the names
of our family and friends;

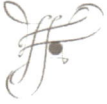

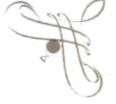

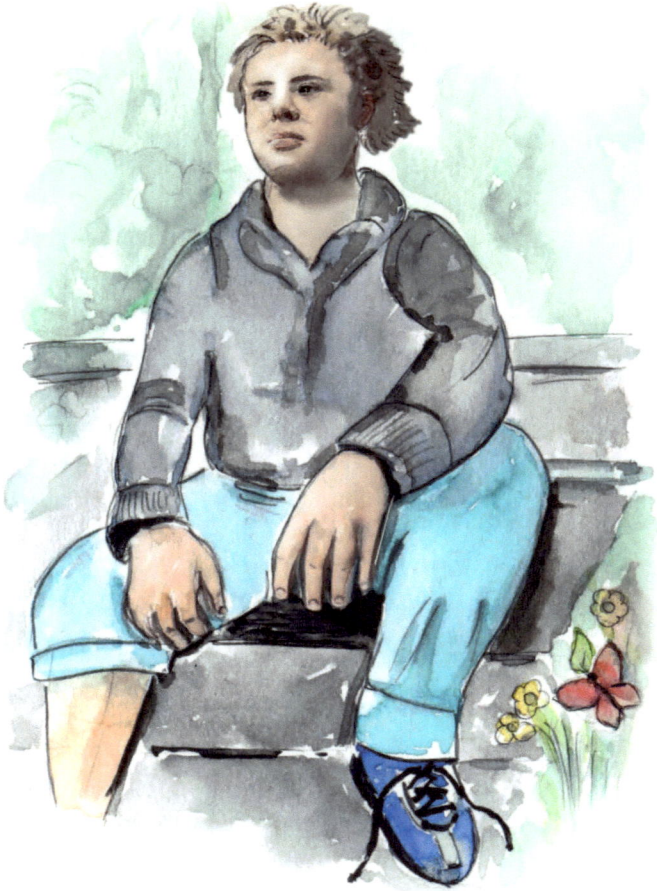

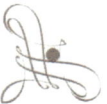

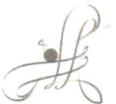

or even how to take care
of ourselves.

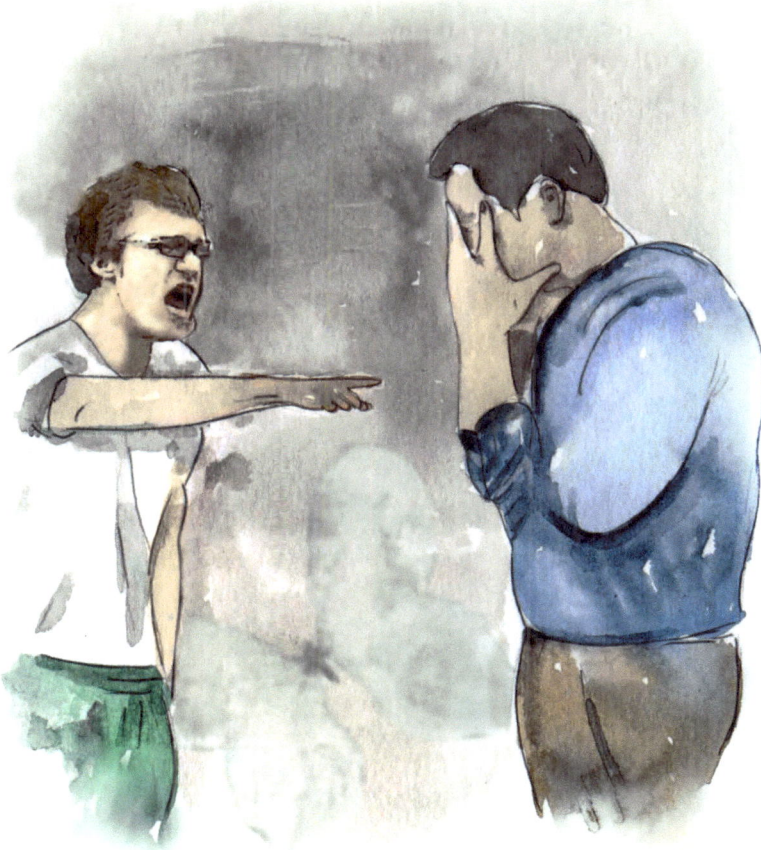

We may forget how to use
our manners even with the
most important people in our lives.

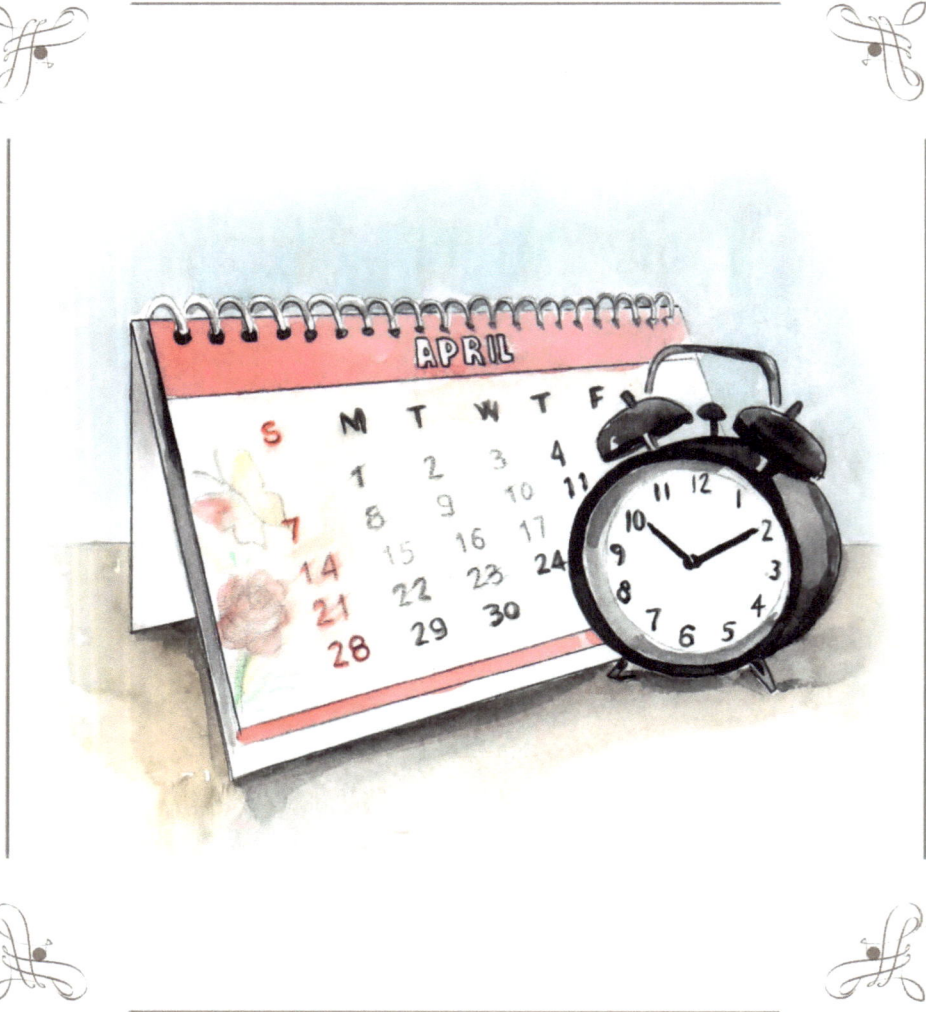

It's difficult to know
how quickly our picture
memories will fade.

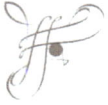

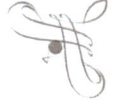

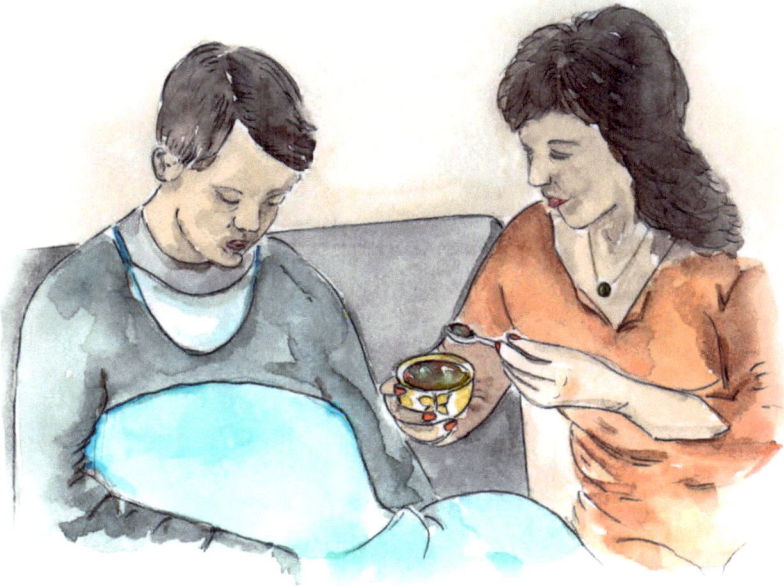

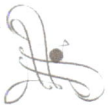

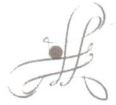

We do know the picture memories
will keep fading and
it will get harder and harder
to take care of ourselves.

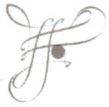

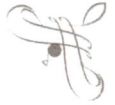

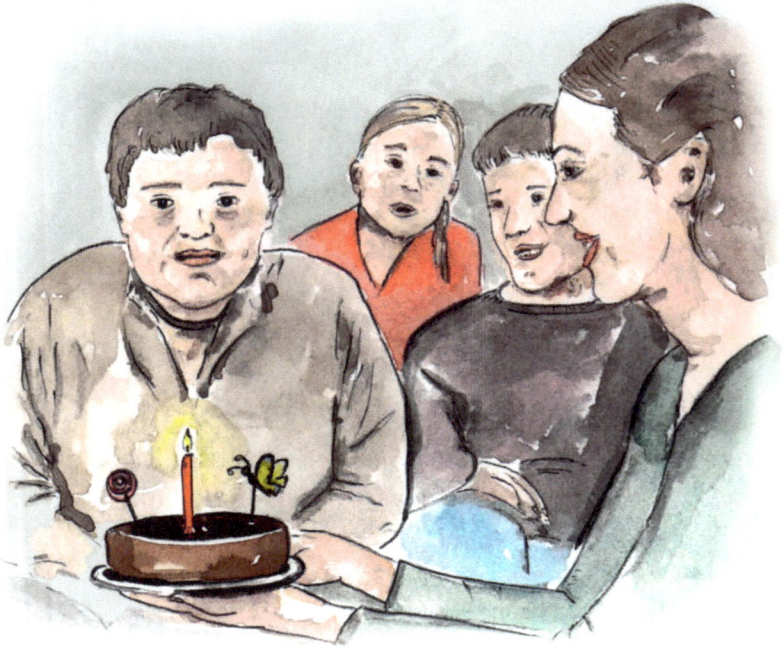

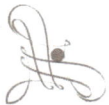

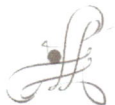

Through all of this,
we will still be able to feel
the love and kindness
from our family and friends.

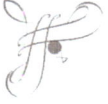

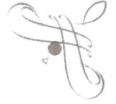

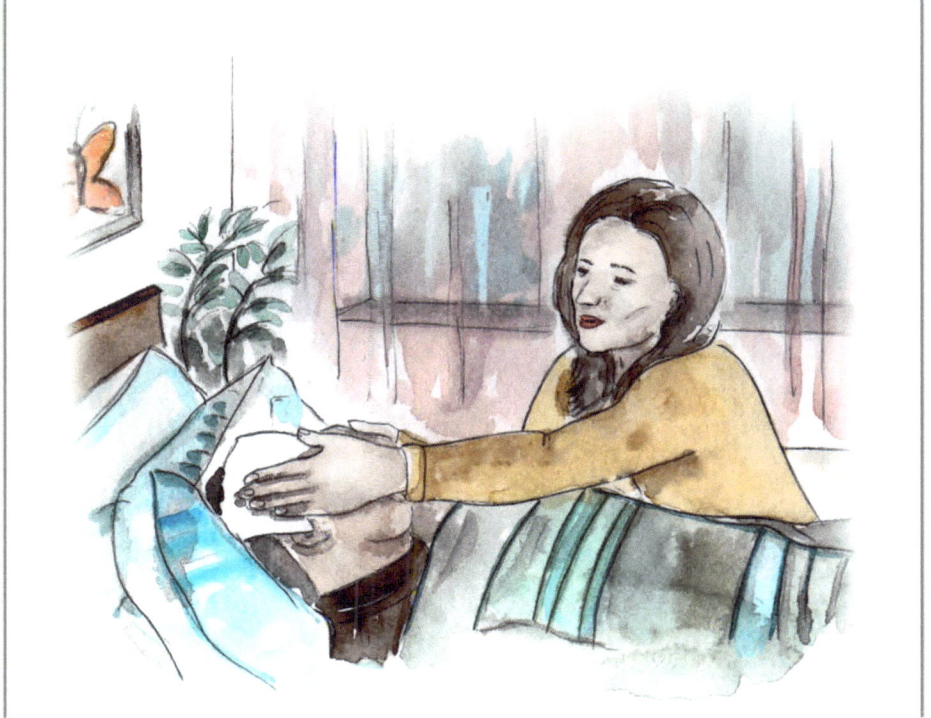

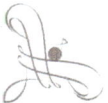

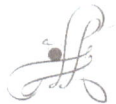

We will count on them
to take care of us
the best way possible.

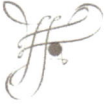

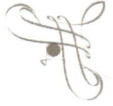

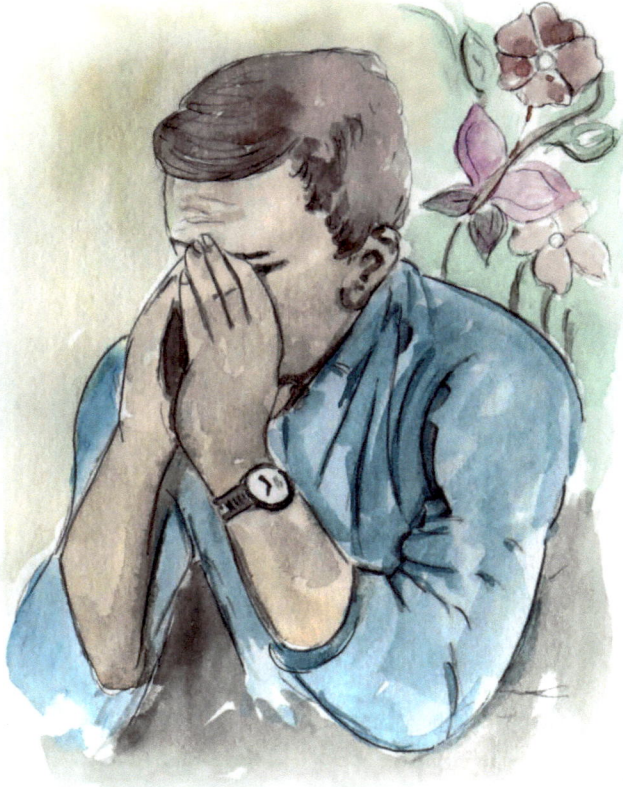

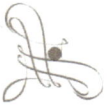

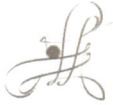

For people in our lives
who help us every day, it can
be really hard to watch as our
picture memories fade.

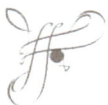

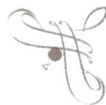

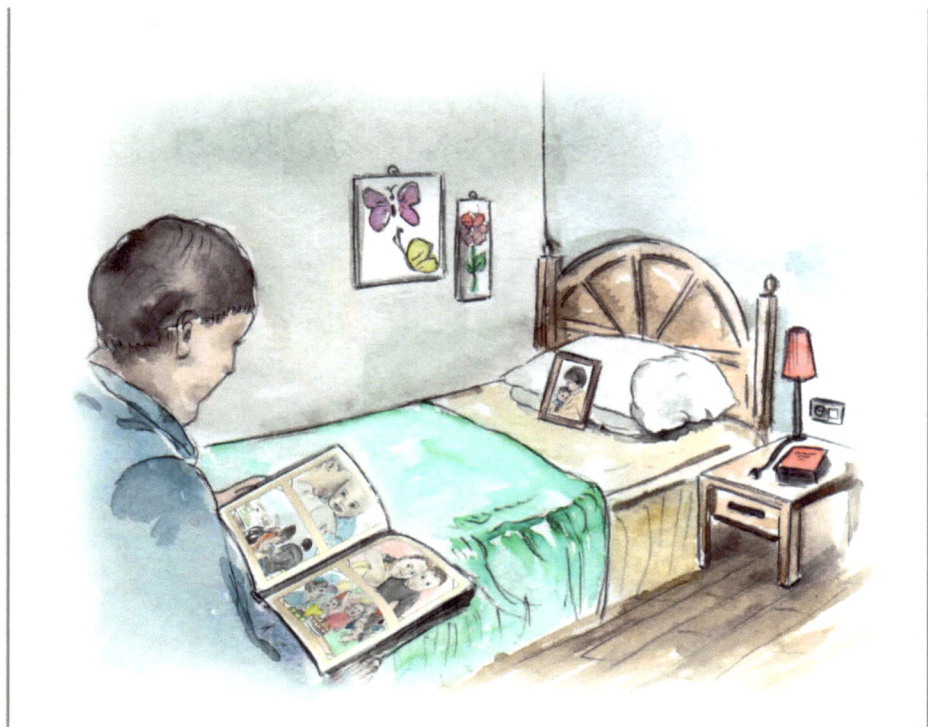

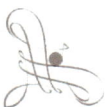

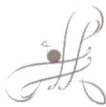

Our caregivers, family and friends
will have their own picture memories of our
times together. They will cherish them
for the rest of their lives.

Did you find the butterfly
in every illustration?

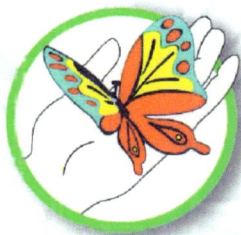

Why the butterfly?

We use the butterfly for our logos because of "The Butterfly Effect." The meaning comes from a 1972 talk given by Edward Lorenz to the American Association for the Advancement of Science describing the chaos theory titled, "Does The Flap Of A Butterfly's Wings In Brazil Set Off A Tornado In Texas." In other words, the ripples of a very small change can make a huge difference down the road.

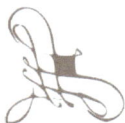

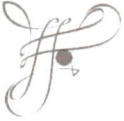

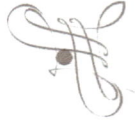

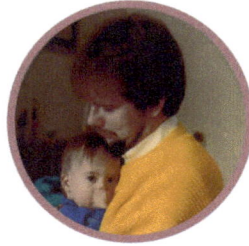

THE INSPIRATION

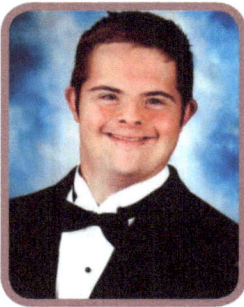

Clayton Lee Henderson, III – Trey – was the inspiration for Henderson Haven, Inc., the organization his parents founded dedicated to ensuring everyone is given the opportunity to live a life of true choice and community inclusion. Encouraged by his family to never give up or say, "I can't", he has always served as an inspiration to others to not give up or settle.

After fighting for his right to participate in the public-school system without being segregated or held back, his parents then stepped aside and let him take the lead. He not only participated in regular classes such as Drivers Ed, he was also involved in extra curricular activities like drama and cheering. He was elected Homecoming King and Most School Spirted by the student body.

After serving on the varsity cheer team for 2 years, he served as the school mascot, Slash, his senior year and found his love for the mascot business. After high school he auditioned for Harriet, The University of North Florida's mascot side kick, and made it. He served in that capacity for a year. He also turned his passion into a vocational skill wearing costumes for local businesses including as the Easter Bunny for the local mall.

Trey continues to work hard to retain the freedom he's become accustomed to. While being diagnosed with dementia has presented new challenges and needed additional supports, he will always be the lead in his life's decisions.

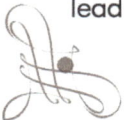

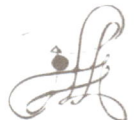

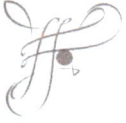

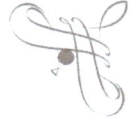

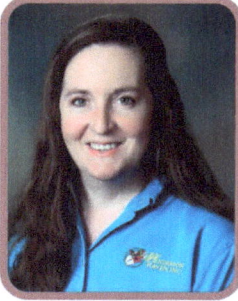

Sherri Henderson founded Henderson Haven, Inc. with her husband, Lee, when families began seeking her advice on providing their children with the same opportunities Trey has had in his life. Always believing that any individual has the capacity to live on their terms regardless of their perceived abilities, she has always fought both personally and professionally to help ensure those rights for all. When informed of Trey's diagnoses and being confronted by him with questions about what it meant, she began to look for tools to help give him an explanation. While she was able to find several publications to help explain Alzheimer's to others as it pertained to family members or loved ones, there was nothing to help explain the condition on a first-person basis and help them understand the symptoms they would be facing. Always taking such challenges personally and believing that this would be a growing need as those with special needs continued to reach higher age milestones, this book is her solution.

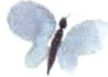

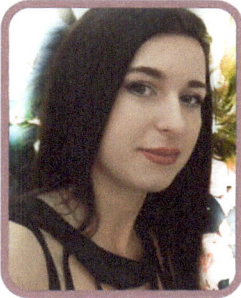

Ani Barmashi lives in Tirana, Albania where she studied architecture for 5 years at Polytechnic University. Having a love of drawing and illustrating all her life, she now operates her own studio specializing in architectural drawing but also works in book, magazine and website illustration. Ani answered a worldwide call Henderson Haven put out to find the perfect illustrator for this project and was chosen out of over 100 candidates because of her obvious talent and her feel for what they were working to accomplish. Henderson Haven is very pleased and honored she joined with them on this project.
Ani can be reached at anibarmashi@gmail.com

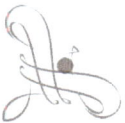

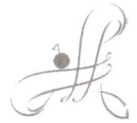

HENDERSON HAVEN, INC.
Independence Through Creativity

METAMORPHOSES
Changing Our Lives for the Better - Together

Free 2 Be Me
REAL life skills for a REAL life

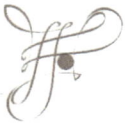

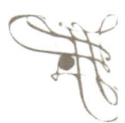

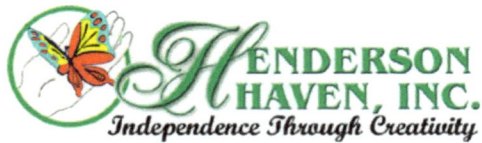

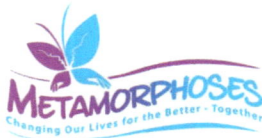

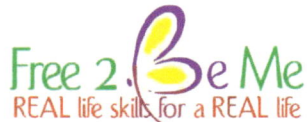

Founded in 2003 by Lee and Sherri Henderson, Henderson Haven, Inc's. non-profit services continue to help ensure a self-determined life and community inclusion for all. Presuming competence in everyone, the staff of Henderson Haven assist those they serve reach their full potential. With services ranging from pre-school, private school, transition, to community supports, Henderson Haven continues to assist everyone in living the lives we all take for granted. For more information or to donate: www.HendersonHaven.org

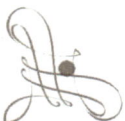

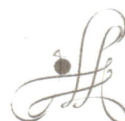

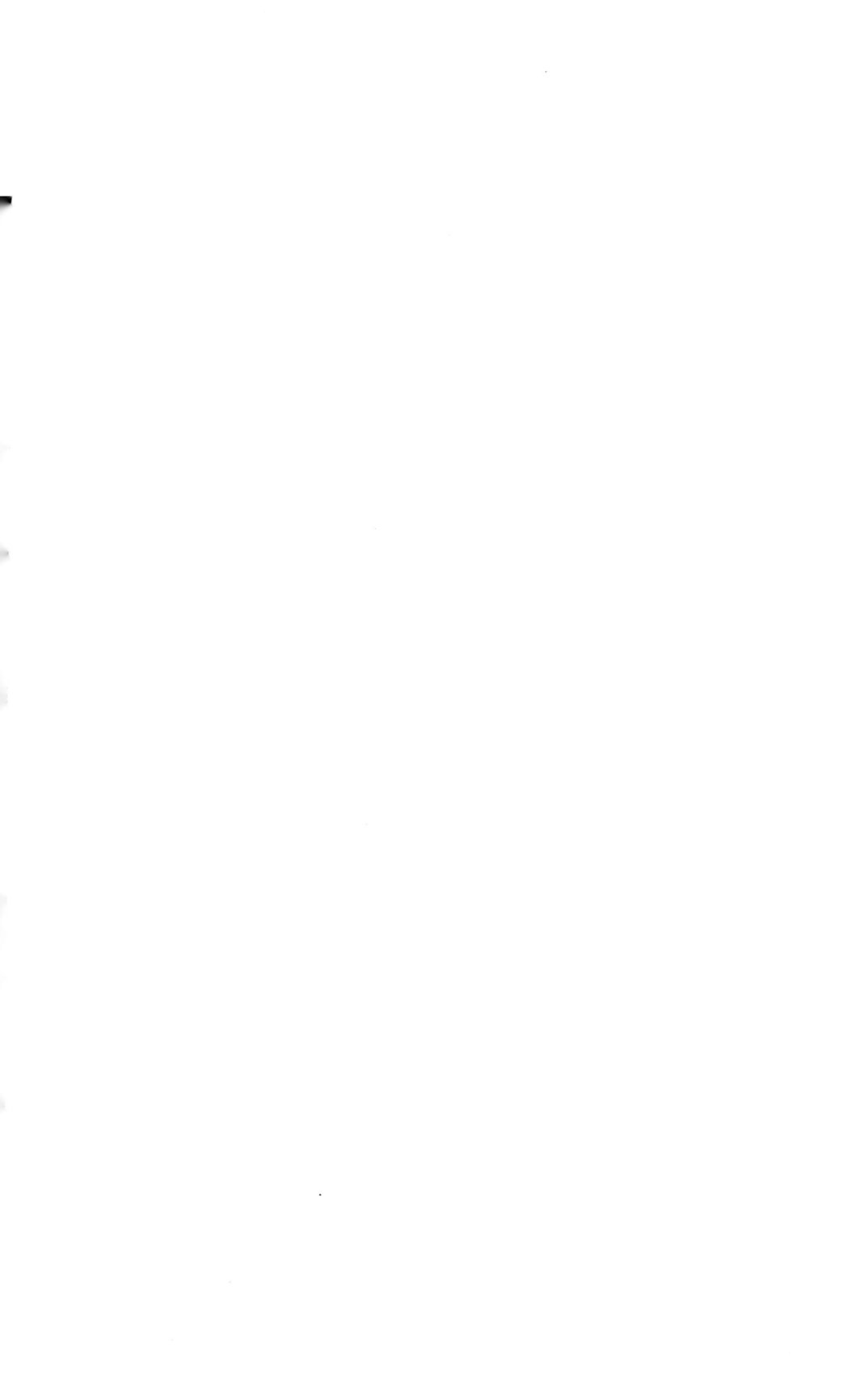

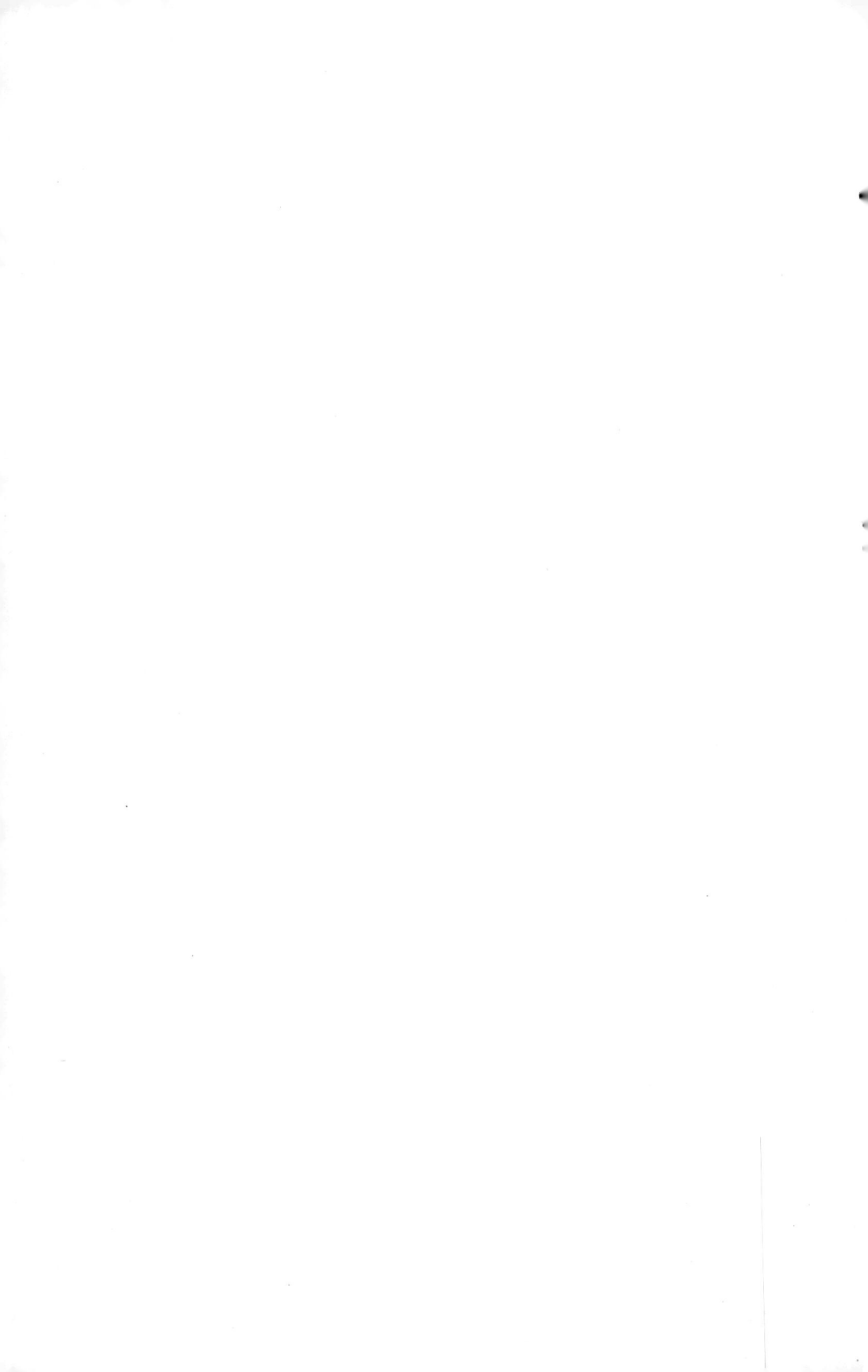